MW01289763

Birthing Freedom

How I Learned to
Relax + Have a Baby

(After the Nightmare "Natural" Birth
of My Firstborn)

Amanda Grace Harrison

Get free videos, resources, and a printable checklist of the exact steps I took to have a fun + easy labor at:

LoveBirthing.co

Disclaimer: This book does not offer medical advice. If you have any concerns with your pregnancy and/or birth, please contact your care provider. I love talking about pregnancy, birth, and motherhood. I support you in having a birth experience that you'll absolutely LOVE. Please always talk to your care provider when making any decisions about your pregnancy and birth. And always choose your care provider wisely.

To my brilliant husband Ian
for his affectionate love, epic support, and
inappropriate humor

To my amazing children
Ben, Elizabeth, and Freedom
for making life magical

To birthing women everywhere

To YOU
for picking up this book and therefore becoming
a part of the LoveBirthing Revolution

Table of Contents

Introduction   1

What this book is NOT   3

Chapter 1. Lost and Confused
    in a Pregnant Sea   5

Chapter 2. Bradley Method Classes (a.k.a. Pain
    Management + Why to Avoid It)   11

Chapter 3. Choosing Our Birthing Center
    (More of What NOT to Do)   14

Chapter 4. Ben's Birth
    (a.k.a. Fighting Against Nature)   17

Chapter 5. The Afterbirth   22

Chapter 6. An Angel Named Freedom   26

Chapter 7. A Different Kind of Pregnancy   30

Chapter 8. Birthing with Dolphins
    (or the Next Best Thing)   34

Chapter 9. Passing through the Ring of Fire   41

Chapter 10. Perfectly Imperfect Timing   45

Chapter 11. My Fun Secret Labor   48

Chapter 12. Just the Two of Us   53

Chapter 13. The Birth of Elizabeth Maude   57

Chapter 14. The Afterbirth II   **61**

Chapter 15. Passing It On   **66**

Chapter 16. Baby #3   **69**

Chapter 17. Birthing Freedom   **73**

Appendix 1.
    What *IS* the Partner's Role Then?   **77**

Appendix 2. Oversupply + What NOT to Do
    with Early Breastfeeding   **79**

Bonus Chapter: Orgasmic Birth/Get Yours Now
    (OB/GYN)   **83**

About the Author   **87**

Introduction

"It's the most pain you'll ever experience, but it's so worth it."

Not exactly the most comforting birthing mantra, eh?

Those are the words my well-intentioned mother repeated over and over throughout the years.

They echoed in my mind, worked their way into my being, and eventually became my truth.

That is, *until* I worked my ass off to **change that old story** and find a completely different way of experiencing birth.

Perhaps you've heard something similar.

Maybe you believe that childbirth is naturally, inherently painful.

I'm here to tell you that it isn't.

A wildly different, spectacularly more beautiful, and incomparably fulfilling experience is possible, and I want *that* to be *your* truth.

Most people find my personal story to be more than a little "out there." In fact, it just freaks 'em right out. I write or say the words **"pain-free, *fun* childbirth"** and all they hear is "*freak show.*"

That's cool. I understand. I would've thought the same thing for most of my life.

That's also why, for a long time, I resisted sharing my story at all. I stayed quiet when women talked about birthing--even though I ached to speak my truth--simply because my experience was so radically different from most.

And when I did share even the tiniest inkling of my experience, I would often watch as women's eyes glazed over and took on a hypnotic daze, as if the very concept of painless birthing were so impossible that they couldn't even entertain the idea.

While I could keep waiting forever for "the right time" to share this--when the mainstream public is more open to alternative birthing styles, etc.--I don't want to run the risk of even *one* more woman missing out on this information *if she's ready to hear it now*.

If this book had been available during my first pregnancy, it could have saved me a freight train of pain and suffering. Not only that, but it could have opened up a whole new world of empowerment,

independence,

spiritual fulfillment,

deep inner peace,

confidence,

strength,

and a true initiation into genuine motherhood.

All things I longed for but just couldn't seem to find.

What this book is NOT

This is *not---at all---*a book recommending that *anyone* follow my steps into what's called "free birthing," DIY birth, or unassisted birth (birthing on your own with no medical assistance, no midwife, nada).

That is a path few will be able to take safely, and the call *must* come from within.

However, I do want to offer the priceless treasures I found along the way, the nuggets of pure gold that contributed to making my birthing experiences so ridiculously pleasant. And which have somehow remained completely unknown to most of the population.

Every woman deserves to have a birth experience as good as it can get *for her*.

I hope that by hearing my story, knowing that a woman is fully capable of birthing her own babies without any medical assistance whatsoever, you will be encouraged.

If I did it even without any outside help, then surely *YOU CAN DO IT* with your birthing support team.

May this story contribute to the movement of more and more women around the world beginning to absolutely *love* birthing.

Chapter 1

Lost and Confused in a Pregnant Sea

In my teens and early 20s, self-preservation and aversion to discomfort led me to loathe the idea of birthing. I decided that if I ever did have children of my own, I would either adopt or schedule a C-section. I never wanted to go through what I saw over and over in movies and on TV--the agony, the screaming, the incomparable pain.

But honestly, I had babysat and nannied so much over the years (starting at age 9) that I stopped even *wanting* to have my own children. Birthing styles were a non-issue.

Cut to my late 20s. By then I had moved to Los Angeles and adopted the whole alternative lifestyle, eating super-healthy and into all things "natural." As my family puts it, I "moved to California and became a hippy." I was also married to my best friend and pregnant. Suddenly the nice, neat C-section didn't sound so nice.

My husband's family was from England, where he and his sister were born at home. In the UK, at least at that time, homebirth was just the normal thing to do. And that sounded beautiful to me. Idyllic even. Over time, I had just come to assume that homebirth was what I would do too.

Until one day, relatively early on my pregnancy, when my husband and I went to see a movie. The opening scene depicted a woman in the agony of labor. She writhed about on her four-poster bed, *screaming* for the doctor. As I watched the scene unfold, my heart sank. Giant hot tears streamed unbidden down my cheeks.

Here lay my unavoidable near future. *This is happening.*

The reality of my situation suddenly began to sink in. What was I going to do? I'm not a woman with a high pain tolerance. In fact, **I'm kind of a big baby**. *What was I going to do?!*

The moment the film ended, I made a beeline to the gift shop in the theater lobby and began frantically looking through their collection of books. Completely irrational, I desperately hoped to find something that would help me through this labyrinth of confusion. A guide, a map, a resource-- something. Anything!

Not only did I *not* find anything in the theater gift shop (of course), but I found almost nothing at the local library or even at the giant bookstores. Even at Amazon! Whaaaaat??

All I could find at the time was traditional mainstream pregnancy advice, like *What to Expect When You're Expecting*. That book is basically a hypochondriac's dream-come-true, with every possible complication listed along with what symptoms to look for.

But what I was craving was some kind of spiritual guidance. In fact, those were the search words I used on Google: "spiritual pregnancy." I'd already read all the typical mainstream BabyCenter type of information, but I wanted to find something that would address the deep, deep, foundational, core-of-my-being fears that were gripping me so tightly.

The closest I came to that was the book *Birthing from Within*. This book at least *approached* those deeper fears. The exercises and questions in the book led me deeper into my specific anxieties. The drawing and art exercises helped me to bring my right brain and creative/intuitive sides into the light.

For example, I discovered--when I noticed that I'd drawn a large clock in my birthing room--that I was specifically afraid of feeling rushed during birth. That would turn out to be useful information later in the game. And, unfortunately, a self-fulfilling prophecy.

Without attending a live *Birthing from Within* workshop or class series, the exercises didn't leave me feeling that much better. I believe the rate was $375 at the time for 6 live classes.

I could just see myself and my husband, covered with body paint, feeling very silly and not at all closer to a sense of inner peace. Plus we'd already signed up for Bradley Method classes with the family friend who'd trained my sister-in-law for her daughter's birth, and we only had room for one birth training in our budget.

Next I bought a little book called *Meditations for a Happy Pregnancy*, which I really enjoyed. It had a short reading--connecting with body, soul, and baby--for each week of pregnancy.

I liked that it incorporated not just what the baby was likely getting up to in there or what my body was experiencing, but also ideas for ways to connect with and holistically care for baby and body and prepare for the birth.

I listened to the accompanying guided meditation CD frequently. It helped me feel a little more peaceful, but I still had that nagging feeling.

I bought the book *HypnoBirthing*, read through it, and also used the accompanying guided meditation CD quite a bit. However, again, without attending any live training in the HypnoBirthing method (for financial reasons), I was left with the feeling that it was more of a band-aid than what I really needed--- some kind of surgery to completely remove the giant lump of fear from my heart.

I had a sneaking (and accurate) suspicion that those peaceful vibes would be MUCH more difficult (if not impossible) to conjure up once labor hit.

I also studied the Lamaze Method a little. And I *loved* Rainbeau Mars' *Zen Mama Pregnancy Yoga* DVD--at least this was something I could *do*.

One of my favorite reads was an ebook titled *Ecstatic Birth* by Jinjee and Storm Talifero. This couple had birthed several of their babies at home with no doctor or midwife, and their story intrigued me. I wasn't ready for anything that radical for my first birth, but I tucked the information away for later.

Finally, I read (or at least skimmed) Grantly Dick-Read's book *Childbirth Without Fear*. This book was enormously eye-opening. Dick-Read observed women's birthing habits all over the world. He noticed that in many cultures women experience no pain or discomfort while delivering their babies, while in others birth can be excruciating.

Dick-Read linked the cause of the pain to a societal fear of birthing. He called it the Fear-Tension-Pain cycle. In nature, as in cultures where women experience easy labors, the mother has no fear of labor. She is relaxed during birth and experiences no pain.

However, in cultures where we've been conditioned to believe that birth is dangerous and painful, women feel fear during labor. This fear causes the muscles in our bodies to involuntarily tense, fighting against nature's attempts to release the baby. It also triggers the production of stress hormones, which actually signal the body to stop labor. The result is that the women feel pain and birthing fails to progress.

Unfortunately, "knowing" intellectually that fear and the resulting tension are what causes pain doesn't actually help you be any less afraid. Especially if things start to head south, the pain begins to be unbearable, and you have no idea how to stop being afraid.

But I'm getting ahead of myself. Let's back it up to those birthing classes we'd signed up for.

Chapter 2

Bradley Method Classes

(a.k.a. Pain Management + Why to Avoid It)

I love the people we met at our birthing classes. I also loved how confident it helped me feel about the stages of labor and what to do with a newborn baby.

Another great feature was having to track exactly what I ate every single day and finding out whether I was getting enough protein, Omega-3's, etc. Very helpful stuff.

BUT... and I know I'm going to step on a lot of really well-intentioned, genuinely loving toes here (which makes this so difficult!), but the truth must be told.

I loved our Bradley Method *teacher* and her overall message of empowering women for birth, helping us believe we could truly make it through a "natural" (i.e. drug-free) birth. However, **I am *not* a fan of the Bradley Method** for the following reasons:

1. **Husband as birth coach?!** Whaaaaat?! While you can be a fantastic *cheerleader*

without ever playing football, it would be odd if the *coach* were someone who's never played the game. Husband-as-labor-coach creates a very strange and unnatural dynamic, putting too much pressure on the hubby *and* not providing the support a woman truly needs during this crucial time. [*See "What IS the Partner's Role Then?" in the appendix*].

2. The whole paradigm of the Bradley Method, *not unlike* 99% of the other birthing classes and methods out there, is that it's all based on **Pain Management**. Meaning there is pretty much *definitely going to be pain*, so you want to learn how to "raise your pain tolerance" and stay calm and relaxed *during* the pain.

This is *so* well intentioned and loving (and such a huge improvement over the just-medicate-the-pain-away paradigm) that I have a hard time poo-pooing it, but it is SO poo-poo! It just doesn't leave room for how amazing birth can naturally be for the vast majority of women. It actually strengthens the expectation of pain during birth.

I want to acknowledge the fact that some women do experience health complications that make a natural birth impossible for them. And there may be many instances in which pain management is a very useful tool.

However, a truly normal, truly natural birth (as opposed to what we've come to think of in our culture as "normal"--hard and painful--and "natural"--really just drug-free) is not one of those instances.

Just imagine for a minute that we were all trained in pain management techniques to help us get through sex. It's absurd, right? It would actually create all kinds of fear in us that would actually make sex painful.

If there's pain during sex, it's a sign that something's off. The woman probably just isn't in the right mental space, so her body isn't supplying the lubrication it normally would. But pain management would not be the appropriate solution.

Birthing is much the same. We would never think of pain management when we prepare for sex, and we don't need to for birth prep either. What we do need is to make the choices that set us up for the best birth experience possible.

Chapter 3

Choosing Our Birthing Center

(More of What NOT to Do)

All of my reading and studying had led me to the conclusion that I needed to feel safe, comfortable, and relaxed during labor in order for it to go as smoothly as possible.

This is something that's easily overlooked when a pregnant mama has a busy life and has to be tough and strong on a daily basis.

My husband used to build houses, and the hours, inconsistent money, and lifestyle were extreme sometimes. I had learned to be tough and resilient. And many moms think that's the best way to approach labor.

But what gets us through an ordinary day isn't what helps us have an easy labor. We actually need to get soft, tune in to the subtle messages from our body, and let go. And that requires being in a space and with people that encourage you to completely relax.

In order to ensure that I would be able to feel safe and relaxed, I needed to choose the right location for the birth. But that wasn't as simple as it may sound.

I really wanted to birth at home. It was the natural choice, because I'm one of those women who feel safer at home than at a hospital.

The *problem* was that we didn't *have* our own home at the time. We were living with family. Specifically, an 85-year-old (now 96-year-old) Middle Eastern woman who is a TINY bit of a worrier, meddler, and micromanager.

The thought of Gramma-in-law hovering over me, offering her oh-so-helpful suggestions and asking every 3 minutes if the baby's here or not, was *way* outside of what would help me to feel relaxed during birth.

Hospitals were also out for me, because:

a) We had no insurance, so it would've been expensive. Possibly *extremely* so if any complications arose, which studies show they are more likely to do if you labor and deliver in a hospital setting. And,

b) I'd learned too much about hospital vs. home birth for that to seem like an option worth paying for even if we did have the money.

So our only real option was a birthing center.

The birthing center I chose, while being comfortable and conveniently across the street from a hospital should an emergency arise, had one big problem that I didn't realize until it was too late.

The center had *two* birthing suites with their own beds and hot tubs, but there was *only one midwife* and her assistant. Having backup midwives most likely would have led to me having a very different birthing experience.

But then I wouldn't be here writing this book. And I wouldn't have gone on to work so hard researching and learning the very best ways to do birth the second and third time around. I would have just continued on birthing with midwives and trusting *their* authority. So, c'est la vie.

But why, you may be asking, was it such a huge mistake for me to birth at a one-midwife clinic? Here it comes...

Chapter 4

Ben's Birth

(a.k.a. Fighting Against Nature)

Remember when I mentioned that my biggest fear about labor, as unearthed in the *Birthing from Within* exercises, was that I would feel rushed?

Well, in my attempts to *avoid* that feeling, I purposely waited until morning before heading to the birthing center, even though I'd been having weird labor all night. My hope was that the midwife and her assistant would be well rested and ready to be patient with me.

Ha!

Instead, they had been up all night with the unexpected early labor of the woman who was scheduled for birth the month *after* me. To use some familiar Old Testament language from my Southern Baptist upbringing, "What I feared had come upon me." Job's extremely uncomfortable reality had become my own.

My labor *seemed to be* progressing quickly. I can clearly remember the midwife commenting to her assistant and my hubby that I was going to be one of those super-quick easy labors, and soon we'd all be home resting. That was probably around 9 a.m.

I purposely kept my eyes off the clock all day, so I have no idea exactly what time things happened after that.

I *do* know that at some point (I'm guessing early afternoon at the earliest), the midwife was so exhausted from being up the night before, and my labor was so stalled out, that she ordered me to *just start pushing*.

Even though I wasn't completely dilated, but more like 9cm with a "lip" (swollen edge of the cervix).

And so I did push.

For hours.

It didn't help much at all, and soon we were *all* beyond exhausted, all the blood vessels in my eyes had burst, and it looked like I was going to have to be transferred to the hospital for either a C-section or an episiotomy.

In fact, my midwife threatening exactly that scenario, if I didn't keep pushing, was the only thing that kept me going.

I wasn't about to pay *even more money* for a hospital birth, or allow my body to be sliced open.

Looking back, it seems horrific that a midwife-- someone supposedly dedicated to bringing babies into this world in the gentlest way possible--would threaten a birthing mother with physical pain if she didn't man up and force her baby out quickly enough.

Or maybe that's just my take on it.

[Note: In her defense, my midwife was also a human being, possibly stretched to the limit of how much her body could handle. She did come down with serious flu-like symptoms the day after my son was born, so that's further evidence that she was genuinely giving her all and doing the best she knew how to do.]

Back to the labor, the ordeal of a lifetime, the "most pain I've ever experienced."

Many times I wanted to give up.

Once or twice I prayed that I would just die. As truly awful as it sounds, at that point I honestly didn't even care if I or my unborn child lived or not.

I was dead to any emotion, completely exhausted on every level. I just wanted it to be over. I needed a nap more than I've ever needed a nap in my entire life.

I couldn't even feel the contractions any longer. The midwife had to tell me when she felt one coming on and command me to bear down with any remaining energy I had. Which was practically nothing.

The only comfort I found was from the thought that at least I could finally identify with the suffering of Jesus (again, the Southern Baptist in me).

I also kept repeating to myself the reality that at some point this would all just be a bizarre memory. Sooner or later, that moment that I wanted so badly to get out of would be in my past.

I begged for that time to come.

Only a miracle got us through that day. Well, a miracle *and* a ton of animalesque growling, grunting, and screaming (honestly, I've never heard those sounds come out of any human). *And* the most intense workout of my life--like trying to run a full marathon without ever having done any endurance training.

I was 110% spent.

I'd heard the words, "You're so close! We can see the head!" so many times I was ready to punch my husband, the midwife, *and* her cute assistant if any of them said it again.

My son's head seemed to move one inch forward and then two inches back, and I lost any connection to the moment.

Their well-meaning cheerleading seemed like the cruel taunts of bullies teasing their prey.

But somehow, finally, I held my sweet, wet, wrinkly little bundle. Ben was born at 6:45 that evening, almost 11 hours after we arrived at the clinic.

Not the longest labor I've heard of, by far, but certainly nowhere near the gentlest.

I looked down at my precious tiny little man through bloodshot eyes. My eyelids were swollen almost completely shut from what they call "purple pushing."

I was barely able to hold him against my chest with my trembling and exhausted arms as I repeated over and over, "We did it… we did it… we did it…."

Chapter 5

The Afterbirth

After all that, just when you'd think I deserved a break, the damn placenta didn't want to cooperate.

As I sat there in the birthing tub, the water long since grown cold, my baby far away with hubby and the assistant doing the measurements and all that good stuff, it honestly felt like I had to go through it all again.

My "tender region," ripped to shreds by the unnatural events of the past few hours, could barely stand the thought of *anything* else passing through that area again.

At one point my exhausted midwife actually *tugged* at the umbilical cord. I had no power left to defend myself. I was too weak and delirious. And as soon as the placenta *did* come out, I began to hemorrhage. *A lot.*

The water in the pristine white birthing tub was dark red with blood when I finally stepped out, shivering, and staggered (with help) to the birthing suite bed.

Fortunately, my sweet baby had no trouble latching on, so at least breastfeeding went smoothly--at first [*see the appendix for an important note about "oversupply" and what NOT to do with early breastfeeding*].

We had to leave the birthing center within an hour of the birth (another downside of choosing this particular location). But at least then we were at home in our very own bed.

I remember that whole first week I kept having the sensation that someone was going to come and take the baby way, like his real parents were going to come back and I'd have to hand him over.

Each time I'd remind myself that this was *our* baby and no one else could take him or tell me I was holding him wrong. And each time I'd be flooded with those magical good-feeling hormones.

Good feelings aside, I lost a ton of blood over those first days. I couldn't walk or stand for long, without feeling like I was going to pass out, so I was stuck in bed for almost a month.

I went through a ton of those frozen maxi-pad compresses. And I hurt like hell for a long, long time.

The silver lining is that it gave me lots of time to bond with my little guy (and take literally 3,000 photos the first month alone), freed from any pressure to get up and tidy the house, introduce him to the great outdoors, or catch up on the rest of life.

I did feel very proud of myself for having made it through that unbelievable ordeal. I heavily identified with the Rosie the Riveter posters other natural birthing moms were posting, exclaiming "We Can Do It!"

I'd made it through a very difficult labor, without any medication.

I would never, however, be able to think of my experience as a truly "*natural* birth."

What specific lessons did I learn from this ordeal?

1. **Have a backup midwife or care provider**. It seems obvious, but it wasn't to me at the time, so it bears stating.

2. **Own your own authority**. I can't stress this one enough. Do your research and training ahead of time so you're not relying on anyone else's expertise. Know and stand up for what you want and need. Don't let anyone else take charge of your birth.

3. **Trust your baby, your body, and nature's perfect timing.** *Your body and your baby know exactly what to do.*

4. On a practical note, have high-protein, unsweetened snacks on hand, not just fruit pops, coconut water and protein bars. (I got really tired of sweets and wanted something non-sweet during labor. Even plain walnuts or pumpkin seeds would've been brilliant.)

Chapter 6

An Angel Named Freedom

During the years after Ben's birth, I occasionally came across new information I'd never heard before about birth. One of my favorites was an article by Ingrid Bauer, "Birth As Sheer Pleasure." I found the article online somewhere, but it was originally published in *Midwifery Today* in 2003.

Ingrid, who had also written the book *Diaper Free!*, which I read while pregnant with Ben, wrote the article to tell about her experience of bliss during birth.

> *"Inevitably, in discussions about unassisted or natural birth, the topic of pain-free birth rolls around. When it does, I wonder if striving for a 'pain-free birth' doesn't inadvertently miss the potential beauty of natural birth itself. I don't believe birth is meant to be pain-free--in fact, I believe it's far more than that!* ***I believe, and have experienced, birth to be downright ecstatically, blissfully, orgasmically pleasurable.*** *'Pain-free' doesn't even come close to describing that experience. That's like calling a high sexual union with your mate 'pain-free,' or the most breathtaking*

sunset you've ever seen 'ugly-free.' For I think that as long as we're focusing on getting rid of, or avoiding pain, we're focusing on the wrong area and we're completely missing the point." [emphasis mine]

This concept was revolutionary to me. Painless was one thing; orgasmically pleasurable is something completely different.

A few months after Ben's 2nd birthday, we took a trip to beautiful Santa Barbara, California. While we waited for my husband outside of a shop (because that's much less stressful than trying to keep a toddler tame in a boutique men's clothing store), Ben entertained himself by jumping off of a bench over and over.

A sweet homeless man in a wheelchair, his legs covered with an American flag, stopped to watch. We struck up a conversation, and I learned that the man's name was Freedom. He told me all about his wife and children, whom he'd lost years ago in a car accident.

When my husband eventually joined us, Freedom tearfully encouraged him to enjoy every minute with his family and never take one day for granted. Then he asked my husband if he could kiss my hand. You can't help but adore a sweet, sincerely gallant older gentleman.

After he kissed my hand, Freedom asked, "Did you *know* you're pregnant with a little girl?"

Wow.

Um, no. Didn't know that. It was right about that time that my period was due, so anything was possible. And it would mean that Ben and the baby would be three years apart, which had always been my wish. *And* it would mean we'd have a big brother and a little sister, just like in my own family, so that would be really cool.

Freedom pulled me back out of my future planning when he asked us to name our daughter after his mother, Elizabeth. We politely agreed. Honestly, at the time it all felt just a tad surreal if not bizarre.

"And in another few years, you're gonna have another little man like this one," he added, gesturing to Ben. "And I want you to name him after *me.*"

"Okay, sure. Yeah. We'll do that. Thank you so much, sir. It was lovely meeting you. Have a beautiful day." And away we went.

Over the next few days, I did indeed begin to experience some early pregnancy symptoms. My period never did show up, so I bought a pregnancy test.

Sure enough, Freedom was right. When my husband announced to his family that we were pregnant, he also told them that she was a girl and we were naming her Elizabeth.

I was impressed. Usually *I'm* the hippy, the woo-woo one. But this time hubby had jumped right on board, which meant in a few years we'd actually have a child named Freedom!

Now for the business of pregnancy and birth planning, round two.

Chapter 7

A Different Kind of Pregnancy

After the drama of that first birthing experience, I knew I wanted to birth at home this time. And we were moving into an apartment, so at least I would have *some* modicum of privacy.

Sick and tired

This baby brought morning sickness (or really just "all-day-long sickness") and daily puking, which I don't remember doing *once* during my first pregnancy.

My mom assured me this was because I was pregnant with a girl. She'd been fine with my older brother but then sick as a dog during my stay in the womb.

I was also so exhausted during first trimester this time that I could only lie in bed helplessly, trying to read to Ben or otherwise keep him entertained in our tiny guest room at my sister-in-law's house. We were staying with them for a month while we waited for our apartment down the street to be ready to move into.

My mother-in-law volunteered to come pick Ben up in the mornings and spend a few hours with him at her house. He absolutely adored these special times with Gramma and Granddad, jam-packed with creative activities and the undivided attention that only retired grandparents can offer.

And I of course so appreciated getting to rest guilt-free and not worry about my little guy.

Then I started to develop strange sinus issues, like I had a bad cold or ridiculous allergies. I found that the only way I could breathe at night (without having to wear Breathe Right strips, which do *not* look attractive and are humiliating to accidentally wear to the corner market in the morning when you have to run out quickly for flax milk) was to cut out all dairy and meat.

Which really sucked because I'd grown into the comforting habit of making myself a lovely cheese sandwich on toast with mayo and tomato every day. But I adjusted my diet and found creative new ways to get protein and calcium.

Meditation

Somewhere in the past year or so I'd picked up the semi-regular habit of meditating, and once Ben was out of the house for a few hours a day, that became a regular daily ritual.

Because I knew the benefits of meditation but couldn't bring myself to sit still and just breathe, I bought a meditation CD designed to quickly get you the same results you'd get over decades of traditional meditation. I sat and listened and breathed for an hour a day *every day.* And just let my monkey mind run wild.

The great thing about this meditation system is that you don't have to still your mind. Even if your mind runs around like a squirrel the entire hour, you get the exact same benefits as if you'd done a true monk-worthy meditation. All scientifically proven. Ah, modern technology.

Reading + Resources

Now it was time to begin my birth training in earnest. Without a midwife or other medical professional to rely on, I was going to have to *be* the birthing expert.

I read everything I could get my hands on, from Ina May Gaskin's books to random online medical journals and every forum available for home birthing and unassisted childbirth.

I pulled back out Jinjee and Storm Talifero's e-book *Ecstatic Birth* (the one where they'd birthed their babies at home with no assistance). While I'd casually read it during my first pregnancy, this time I was ready to follow their advice and learn from their example.

I re-read Grantly Dick-Read's book *Childbirth Without Fear*, cover to cover, this time being careful not to skim over anything.

And while I still did Rainbeau Mars' *ZenMama* Prenatal Yoga DVD, as well as some other DVD's I'd brought home from the library, my absolute favorite pregnancy workout came from the DVD I ordered from Amazon--*Amira's Bellydancing and Yoga for Pregnancy*.

That video not only provided a great prenatal workout, but it also gave me the hope of a smoother labor this time around, thanks to the special section on simple dance moves to use during labor and for specific pregnancy needs like turning a breech baby.

There was still a huge piece missing, which I would find when I went in search of a very different kind of birthing experience...

Chapter 8

Birthing with Dolphins

(or the Next Best Thing)

Right around Ben's 2nd birthday, we'd been living in Hawaii for a few months while my hubby worked on a solar energy project. While there, I had read several books about dolphins, including a few stories that were more than a little "out there."

They described healing encounters with dolphins as well as actual dolphin-assisted water births in the ocean. Being a dolphin lover, I found the idea fascinating. I even dreamt about dolphins every night for a while.

Back in L.A. and pregnant, I contacted one of the authors, who I knew to be involved in arranging dolphin-assisted births in the warm, shallow waters near her home on the Big Island.

While I really wanted to get back to Hawaii to experience that for myself, I couldn't quite coordinate that on our family's budget. So I asked her if she knew of anyone who was involved with dolphin-assisted birthing in California. While I knew the water was probably too cold for me, it was a trail I just had to follow.

The author replied that she didn't know if anyone was doing that sort of thing in California, but if anyone *would* know, it would be Elena Tonetti-Vladimirova.

Elena had been involved with alternative birth practices since 1982, when she began studying under Igor Charkovsky, the Russian water birth pioneer. For years she worked at a birth camp at the Black Sea where babies were born in the presence of wild dolphins.

As it turned out, Elena was no longer involved in any kind of dolphin-related birthing. However, she had made a documentary about conscious birth, called *Birth As We Know It.*

I watched the 10-minute promo for the movie over and over until finally I found a special running on the DVD--buy one, get one free. I ordered two copies immediately.

The first time I watched the film, I went through nearly an entire box of Kleenex. It explained so much about why my first birthing experience had gone so far off track. It showed so many examples of what gentle, conscious birthing can be like. It made me hungry for more.

I watched the film again, this time with the director's commentary turned on, and learned even more. I wrote my favorite quotes in a journal and read them over and over.

I watched Elena's film almost every single day for the rest of the pregnancy, sometimes twice.

One of my favorite stories from the film is of a little girl who had a traumatic birth experience and only ever drew with gray or black crayons. That little girl watched the film every day, putting it in the VCR herself (this was obviously back in the good ol' days).

One day, after she popped the video out, she announced to her mom, "That's how *I* was born!" And from that day forward, she used every color in the crayon box.

Ben loved watching the movie with me. There was gorgeous footage of babies and children swimming with dolphins. But his favorite part was what he called "The Happy Girl."

Amber Hartnell, a close friend of Elena's, unexpectedly experienced a full orgasm while birthing her son. The footage of her birth, which just looks like a pregnant woman smiling in a hot tub and riding mild waves of drunken pleasure, is featured in both *Birth As We Know It* and the documentary *Orgasmic Birth*.

Whenever I watched the DVD, Ben would request the scene with the happy girl. I loved watching that scene as well, because her birth was the only one that looked not only painless, but easy and pleasurable as well. I wanted my next birth to be as close to that as possible.

So while I wasn't to get the dolphin birth of my dreams, I did get introduced to the extraordinary Elena Tonetti. I found out that she'd also developed the Birth Into Being Method, a powerful shortcut to healing our own birth trauma by creating new reference points in the nervous system. As it turned out, Elena would be leading a workshop at her home in Chico, California the month before my baby was due.

The decision of whether or not to make the 9+-hour drive (including pit stops) up to Chico was not an easy one.

I've been a consistently indecisive, self-doubting person for much of my life. I kept second-guessing, worrying about whether it would actually be worth the time, money, and stress of the long road trip with our 2-year-old.

I would also be leaving Ben with his papa all day long for two full days, seeing them only in the evening. I'd never been away from Ben for more than a few hours in his entire life. It was such a difficult decision, and I vacillated more times than I can count.

Would it actually help? Or would I be filled with regret and feel stupid for dragging my family on a hair-brained adventure?

In the end, the workshop won. We made the long journey, despite multiple "threshold guardians" crossing our path along the way. So many times I was tempted to turn back, to take the complications as a sign that I'd made the wrong decision. I'm so glad we kept going.

Meeting Elena in person was healing in itself. It was like spending time in the presence of Mother Nature herself.

And it was beautiful to be surrounded by a whole group of other adults dedicated to the pursuit of a more conscious way of life. The workshop was profoundly life-altering for me.

And at the end of the 2-day workshop, just as everyone was saying goodbye, I asked Elena if I could have a private word with her.

I wanted to know if she thought I was insane to be planning an unassisted home birth. Now that she'd spent two full days with me, hearing lots of my inner mess and witnessing what I thought of as my chaotic energy, I thought she'd have a decent idea of what I could manage.

Elena lovingly took me by the hand and said something like, "Every mama cat knows how to birth her kittens. And you're no different."

I so wanted to believe that what she said was true, but I still felt as if I were uniquely messed up.

Elena blasted right through that dark cloud with one question: "Didn't you burn through an awful lot of karma during your last birth?"

I wasn't a huge believer in karma, but her words made a lot of sense to me. Not to mention the fact that they were coming right out of the mouth of Mother Nature.

Elena did recommend that I not get attached to *any* particular outcome for my upcoming birth, but stay present and conscious and flexible. She advised me to have a midwife on hand or at least on call, in case anything should come up.

While I would have loved to have done that, just to calm my own fears and have someone else to rely on, our finances just wouldn't allow it.

When we got back to LA I contacted several midwives to see if anyone would be willing to be a "backup plan," but none of them responded favorably. I didn't blame them.

Unassisted birth really is a big risk, and who wants their name or their reputation to be on the line for someone they don't even know?

Chapter 9

Passing through the Ring of Fire

Those last few weeks before Elizabeth was born were intense and emotional.

I was up nearly every night researching past midnight, reading every thread on the unassisted birthing forums, every birthing story I could get my eyes on. I wanted to be prepared for every possible complication.

I was completely terrified, way more so than I'd been with the first pregnancy, because this time I honestly thought I might die. Or end up in prison.

The laws around home birth are so gray, and I knew I was taking a huge risk. If it hadn't been on the plane of a spiritual commitment, and absolutely sure-in-my-bones that I *had to* do this, I would have backed out.

Or maybe, lest I sound too spiritual and holy, it was just the fact that we had no money for a midwife, and no insurance for a hospital birth. My options were limited.

Two weeks before my due date, we drove out to Vegas to celebrate the birthday of one of our dearest friends. Part of the festivities included attending Cirque du Soleil's show "The Beatles LOVE" What an incredibly beautiful experience. I cried throughout pretty much the entire show.

Some of the lyrics were comforting and inspiring, like, "All You Need is Love." But then there was the climactic "A Day in the Life," followed by "Hey Jude."

[*Spoiler alert! Don't read the next paragraph if you haven't seen the show and would be bugged to have any of the story given away*].

When the young boy, who looked an awful lot like my son with his mop of blond hair, lost his mother in a car accident, I took that very personally. While "Hey Jude" is meant to bring hope in a time of sorrow, I felt so completely how traumatic it would be for little Ben if I were to die during birth.

From that moment forward, I began to think there was a really good chance I would die. And yet I just couldn't change paths.

One quote brought me hope and comfort during that time. It was a passage from the book *Women of the Light*, edited by Kenneth Ray Stubbs, Ph.D. Elena had been given a box filled with copies of that book, and she gave a free copy to everyone who attended her workshop.

In the particular passage that spoke to me, from the chapter entitled, "The Meditation Teacher," a woman is sharing her story of meeting a *sannyasin* (an Indian term meaning a person committed to the spiritual path). He said to her:

> *"To become a sannyasin is to enter into the flames of love. It is dangerous, and yet it is incredibly beautiful. Only danger is beautiful because only danger brings you to moments of joy and ecstasy. Only in danger does your life take on a kind of intensity. Then everything is intense: joy is intense, sadness is intense. All is fire. If you can pass through the fire of love, it consumes you--it consumes all that can be consumed. In the end, only a pure consciousness is left behind. So let it become your very path!"*

My life certainly had taken on a kind of *intensity*, to say the least. And what I was planning was indeed considered *dangerous* by most. "Passing through the fire" felt like a pretty accurate description of what I was experiencing.

It was nothing short of a spiritual ordeal. The ultimate test of my faith. I had no one at all to rely on beyond God, my body, and myself.

Chapter 10

Perfectly Imperfect Timing

As if matters weren't complicated enough, the baby didn't arrive quite when I expected. Unlike my son, who came a few days early, my daughter decided to hang out in the womb for a full 42 weeks (that's two whole weeks past our due date).

As we got further and further past baby's expected arrival, I had new concerns. I jumped on the online pregnancy forums and researched the heck out of the dangers of going too long.

"Is this okay?" I knew the due date was only a rough estimate, but how far past the due date is safe and still considered "normal"?

"Am I crazy?" This thought was never far from my mind, but I was able to seek reassurance from the hundreds if not thousands of moms, midwives, and doulas available on the forums.

It turned out that two weeks past the due date was perfectly normal and fine. But that didn't help with the fact that, because the birth was going to happen so much later than expected, our timing was completely thrown off.

My mom had planned on arriving from the East Coast a week and a half after the baby. Now she was going to be there, staying in our apartment, *when the baby was born*. That sounds like a good thing, right? In this case, not so much.

While I adore my mom, she was definitely not one of my greatest supporters in the whole unassisted aspect of the birth. Mom had worked in hospital administration for more than twenty years, so most of her friends were nurses and doctors. They filled her head full of all kinds of worries and fears.

In their defense, they really couldn't help it. They'd witnessed so many complications and traumatic births in the hospital setting that an out-of-hospital unassisted birth must have sounded about as smart as attempting brain surgery at home.

The problem was that I'd learned from Elena that it's super important for the mom to be completely at ease during labor and birth. That she not have anyone in "the birthing field" that causes her stress. And that if something were to cause her undue stress during labor, it would most likely lead to complications.

We couldn't afford complications.

And yet, we couldn't control the situation either. There was nowhere else for Mama to stay, and there was no rushing a truly "natural" birth.

We would just have to trust and wait. And we wouldn't be let down.

Chapter 11

My Fun Secret Labor

Mom arrived in town, and our baby girl showed no signs of wanting to leave the warmth and comfort of her cozy little home in my womb.

We did normal mom's-in-town kind of activities and kept thinking any minute now I'd go into labor. After a few days, Mom actually started to worry that she was going to miss the baby completely.

But finally, only a few days before the end of her visit, I began to have those Braxton-Hicks surges that let me know we were on our way.

Of course I didn't *tell* Mama about them.

It was about 7pm when I realized what was happening, and I pulled my husband aside while Mama was playing with Ben in his playroom.

I didn't even have to say anything. He could tell by my energy, and the fact that I was about to tell him a secret.

"Is this it?" he asked, matching my excitement.

We both agreed not to tell my mom or Ben. Best to just keep it between us and let labor play out on its own. It could take a couple days of these gentle contractions anyway, and there was no need to get them all hopped up about it.

The last thing I wanted was my mom to be squeezing me with excited tears every 5 minutes or constantly checking in to see how labor was progressing.

So instead I just went about ordinary life as if nothing were happening. Whenever a surge would come over me, I would just gently sway or bounce for a minute or so until it passed.

The movements were a little like a mom swaying and bouncing to keep her baby calm as she waits in line at the grocery store. Fortunately, I'd been doing these kinds of movements for the last few months of pregnancy, so nothing seemed odd about it.

Mom never had a clue!

The only hiccup came during the night. A week before baby was due, we had rented a birthing tub. It took up the entire bedroom of our tiny apartment, so we had to move our mattress out to the living room.

That was better anyway, since we had a window A/C unit out there, and not in the bedroom. September in Los Angeles can be ridiculously hot, and trying to get comfortable enough to sleep when you're more than 9 months pregnant is hard enough without the heat factor.

But it also meant that all four of us were sleeping in the living room together--mom on the sofa and the rest of us on the mattress on the floor. One big happy slumber party.

For the first part of the night, I just got up whenever I felt a surge coming. They were far enough apart still (10 to 25 minutes) that I still got a little rest between contractions. Little cat naps. And Mama just kept snoring right through it all (or as her loving friend calls it, "purring").

However, I finally started to get really sleepy, so I lay down in bed. I didn't feel like getting up when the next contraction began, so I just stayed in bed and hoped to do breathing exercises to get through it.

Ouch!

That one contraction *without* movement or dancing showed me all too vividly just how powerful the dancing was for keeping that energy moving through me.

So when the next one came along, I popped up out of bed and was happy to do some swaying and bouncing in the hallway, make another trip to the toilet, and get back to bed. Fortunately, labor slowed down a lot overnight, and I was able to get some serious sleep.

The next morning, I was back to doing the movements whenever a surge came, and between the movements and some breath work, I was able to carry on without Mama suspecting anything.

In fact, I even attempted to have a serious conversation with her out on the front porch that morning to work out some of the tension that still lingered between us.

We'd gone through so many difficult years together when I was a teenager. I just wanted to clear the air (and the birthing field, following Elena's guidance) and make complete peace.

Neither of us had the language to communicate what we really wanted to say, so it didn't go very deep. But at least we tried.

I stood up and gently swayed and bounced as we chatted. The surges kept rolling through every 7 to 15 minutes.

And then it was time for Mama and Ben to go to a late lunch at Great Gramma's favorite Mediterranean restaurant. Thank God we had planned this one in advance, and it "just happened" to be epically perfect timing.

We had no idea how useful it would be to have them out of the house at precisely this moment.

Chapter 12

Just the Two of Us

As soon as they'd driven away, Ian and I looked at each other excitedly.

I offered two suggestions: we could either go on one last relaxing date--a walk at Descanso Gardens, the gorgeous park near our home--or we could just concentrate on serious labor and let the baby come.

"Let's have a baby!" he answered. We were ready to meet our little girl.

As soon as we'd made that decision, my body responded powerfully. A much stronger surge came over me, and active labor began in earnest. I knew we'd made the right decision.

We turned the belly dancing video on, along with the labor playlist I'd spent hours agonizing over, and I pulled out my **birthing mantras**.

For this birth, one of my favorites was:

"Don't just get *through* it, get INTO it!"

That's exactly what I intended to do.

My other favorite, which came in SO handy, and I believe was largely responsible for the paradigm shift that enabled me to really stay in pleasure and not experience any pain during labor or delivery, was:

"This is an INTENSE SENSATION."

I got that one from Ingrid Bauer, one of my birthing sheroes, as you may recall. In her legendary article "Birth As Sheer Pleasure" (the one originally published in *Midwifery Today* in 2003, where she compared "pain-free birth" to an "ugly-free" sunset), she said that during labor, the words "This is only sensation" came very clearly, out of nowhere, into her awareness.

I remembered from my first birth experience just how intense the "sensations" could be, so I turned that into a mantra that would re-frame what could otherwise be translated as pain. And it worked!

Labor progressed quickly. I danced through each contraction (which I continued to call "surges," because I like that name better).

I could actually feel the uterine muscles doing what I'd learned they do. The outer, vertical layer was gently pulling up like a hot air balloon in order to open the horizontal inner layer to release the baby. It felt amazing.

After maybe an hour I made one last trip to the toilet and then climbed into the birthing tub.

I remember my hubby pulling up a chair and putting his feet up on the tub. I would later learn that he figured we had several hours to go, based on how slowly our last labor had progressed and the fact that I was so relaxed and calm. He didn't really believe anything was happening yet and wanted to get comfortable.

Right about this time, we heard Ben and my mom come in the front door. My mom was, of course, overjoyed when she saw what was going on. She gave me a tearful squeeze and tried her best to play cool.

Ian went out to the street to say hi to his sister, who had dropped them off, and to get Ben's car seat out of her car.

As soon as he left, I felt a wave of nausea. *"Oh no, am I going to throw up?"* I thought. But just as quickly, the nausea was gone.

And suddenly an enormous wave of energy swept through me. It took over my body and out came an involuntary, "Whooooooooooooaaaa!"

Everything felt completely different.

That's when I realized that split-second of nausea must have been Transition, that stage of labor immediately preceding delivery.

I could feel that the baby's head had moved lower in the birth canal during that contraction.

Mama came back from peeing to see what all the noise had been. "Mom, get Ian. The baby is coming."

She gave me an excited kiss and ran outside to yell to Ian and start calling the family to tell them to pray.

Little did she know just how quickly labor would pass.

Chapter 13

The Birth of Elizabeth Maude

Ian made it back inside just in time for the last two contractions.

He'd heard my big "Whoooooaaaaa!" but since he'd never heard me make that kind of noise before, he'd assumed it was the neighbor kids playing.

He and Ben watched from the side of the tub as the waves washed over me, bringing our baby into the world.

True to what I'd learned about the Fetal Ejection Reflex, I never pushed at all. There were only three big "rushes"--that first one that brought her down into the canal, one that brought her head to crowning, and one that brought her head out.

My body had completely taken over and known exactly what to do.

And also true to what I'd been training for, there was **no pain whatsoever** in the entire labor and delivery process.

The only moment there was any sensation that *could have* been described as "pain" was one nanosecond during that final surge, as the baby's head was passing through.

For one split second, there was a flash of heat so brief that only afterwards could I formulate the thought, *"Oh, that must have been the 'ring of fire.'"* I'd read about the Ring of Fire in lots of places as I prepped for this birth, and it was a great description for it.

With my first birth, I spent so many hours in pushing and straining and fighting against nature that I don't remember much of the actual sensations when he finally came out. I just remember the relief and the exhaustion.

But with this birth I was able to experience *everything*, and that Ring of Fire was actually amazing. While it sounds scary and painful and like something to be avoided, it's so not.

It's just like that quote that had gotten me through the ordeal of pre-birth fear. Passing through the flames of love is dangerous but beautiful. Life-altering in the best way possible.

I remember so clearly feeling her precious little head as we patiently waited for her to turn and pop her shoulders out. It was so soft--the softest thing I'd ever felt, with its extra skin and soft, fine hair covered with vernix (the waxy white substance coating the skin of newborns).

But what were those weird flaps on the side--like some kind of extra tissue or something. Was she deformed? Did some part of my body come out with her that wasn't supposed to?

Then I felt around to the front of her head and found her little nose. That's when it hit me. Silly me, those flaps were her adorable little ears! How precious!

I'll never forget that moment of relief and joy. Sigh. She's normal and healthy. And she has ears!

Sometimes it's the really simple things in life that trip us up. I couldn't stop passing my hand over her head and feeling those adorable little ears.

Her tiny body began to turn inside me. Once she was completely sideways, her body just slipped right out into the water. I ever so slowly brought her up to the surface, letting her feel the water around her.

I placed her immediately on my chest and wrapped her in a warm towel. Holding her head on an angle, I rubbed her back firmly to squeeze out any water that was still in her lungs or nose.

She wriggled and made soft little noises. Our baby girl was here!

Just then, Mom came back in. Of course she was overwhelmed with excitement.

"What?! Oh my goodness! I missed it? She's here! Wow, that was fast!" Tears streamed down her face as she kissed the baby and me. Then she joined Ben in watching me watch the baby, and Ian went to call family and friends to tell them the good news.

Elizabeth latched on right away, and I kept her warm against me, covered in a fluffy towel.

Ben, who would be 3 in just 3 days, was thrilled when we said he could finally climb into the birthing tub. He'd been wanting to swim in it for a couple weeks by that point, but I'd kept him out to keep it clean for the birth.

He stripped off his clothes and climbed in to get a closer look at his new little sister. However, when he tired of watching the tiny wriggling baby and wanted to splash around in the water, we instead sent him to dry off and get dressed.

More family and friends had arrived by then, and Ben and my mom went out to be with them in the living room.

Chapter 14

The Afterbirth II

After the family and friends had come in for a quiet peek at the baby and returned to the living room, Ian and I were finally alone with the baby for some quiet bonding time. We enjoyed the post-birth bliss for as long as we could.

I lasted longer than Ian, who wanted to give me some 1-on-1 time with baby while he attended to our guests.

The placenta also had yet to be delivered. So in the tub I stayed, just basking in the glow of birth, adoring my new little wonder.

Eventually I began to get uncomfortable. Birthing tubs really aren't designed for lounging and nursing your newborn.

The hitch was that we'd decided to attempt a Lotus Birth. That's where you leave the umbilical cord uncut after birth. The placenta remains attached to the baby until it naturally dries up and falls off on its own, 3-10 days after birth.

Looking back, that sounds absolutely absurd that I even thought I was remotely the kind of person who could handle that kind of extra work. You have to protect the placenta from rotting by wrapping it in herbs and changing the cloth around it frequently.

It's just a whole lot of extra hassle for what is essentially a really beautiful *idea.*

"Let's do it all-natural," we idealists say. Yeah, but life in the modern world isn't all natural. And as a *New York Post* article on the subject put it, "Think caring for a newborn is hard? Try a newborn that's still attached to its placenta!"

In this case, the umbilical cord was of course still attached to the placenta that was still inside me.

It can take anywhere from 10 minutes to an hour on average for the placenta to be delivered, and some cases go much longer than that. So as I was sitting there holding my precious girl, the cord (which was only maybe 20 inches long), was tugging ever-so-slightly *down there.* It wasn't a pleasant effect.

That attachment also meant no one else could hold the baby until I'd delivered the placenta, or at least not without causing me extra discomfort. So I waited and waited, for more than an hour after the birth, for the placenta to be delivered.

At one point, I called out to Ian. Could he please google the situation and find out what we should do? He surprised me with his response.

Hubby replied that I'd trusted God for every detail of this birth so far--why start doubting and taking matters into my own hands now?

He was right. I thought back to how perfectly everything had worked out with the timing of my mom and Ben being gone for labor but showing up just in time for the birth.

I couldn't have planned that if I tried.

The placenta did, indeed, finally eject itself. Mostly. The fibrous ends were still attached or otherwise stuck inside me. I didn't dare tug and risk all that crazy hemorrhaging again. So again I waited. And waited.

Meanwhile I was starting to get really pruny and tired of soaking in the uncomfortable tub. So we agreed I would get out and dry off, no matter how awkward that would be with a placenta hanging out of me.

It would require a lot of outside help. Someone would need to hold the baby, and I'd need to hold the placenta (really a two-hand job to be safe) while somehow climbing out of the tub and drying off.

Fortunately, the minute I stood up, the placenta completely detached. Gravity was just the thing it needed. We were able to put the placenta in a bowl and finally take the baby out to the living room while I went to the bathroom to get cleaned up and dressed.

Hours later, after Ben had jumped on the bed and jostled the placenta bowl one too many times, we decided the lotus birth had gone on long enough.

Ben was beyond excited to help cut the cord, and we were relieved to finally have the freedom to move the baby around without that giant alien organ.

In hindsight, what about this birth would I do differently?

1. Close the blinds and **dim the lights in the birthing room**. 4:44 pm in September in Los Angeles, in a bedroom with west-facing windows, was ridiculously bright. Poor little newborn. What a shocker that must have been. But my mind was elsewhere. ;)

2. Don't be afraid to *slow it down*. Part of me still felt like faster was better. I wish I'd purposely slowed down and really enjoyed the experience.

3. For a planned unassisted birth, hire a midwife to at least be on call. Financially I don't know how we could have done it, but even just doing prenatal care with a midwife could have saved me a lot of stress over unknowns.

On the flip side, I probably wouldn't have owned my own authority so completely. So while I'm glad I did it totally solo for some reasons, I could have at least called some midwives and gotten some prices on how much prenatal care without delivery would have cost.

Chapter 15

Passing It On

After experiencing the absolute bliss of birthing without pain--not just that, but actually having *fun* during labor--I felt like I'd gotten away with something.

It didn't feel fair. I didn't want to be the only one. In fact, now that I knew what was possible, I wanted every woman everywhere to experience it.

Watching movies that involved birthing scenes became almost unbearable. I wanted to stand up and shout, "It doesn't have to be that way!"

While I wanted to share the secret with others, I found that when I mentioned the concept of pain-free, blissful labor, most people looked at me like I had three heads. I hated it.

After almost three years of wishing I could share the information, I still hadn't really managed to pass the experience on to anyone else. It burned inside me and cried out for expression like a character from a story that's aching to be told.

I started working with an energy coach just for fun. After several months of knowing me and hearing what was important to me, she recommended that I write an article about how to have a fun, painless birth.

So I wrote it all out, including which books, DVDs, mantras, ideas, workshops and websites had had the biggest impact on me and created the most profound difference between birth 1 and birth 2.

When I looked for places to publish the article, however, I found that the magazines I knew would be just the right fit had gone out of print. Hmmmmm. Now what to do.

I sat on the article for a few weeks like a mother hen, trusting that at some point it would be ready for action.

I joined a Meetup group for homebirth enthusiasts and attended one of their events, but none of the moms there were very interested in my story.

I guess it's just too far outside most people's comfort zones. I was starting to feel like an evangelist preaching to a disinterested world.

Finally, one mama-to-be contacted me. She'd read my bio on the homebirth Meetup page and was very intrigued. She'd never heard of a pain-free, blissful birth and wanted to know everything.

I immediately emailed her the article I'd written.

That mama followed every bit of advice I'd outlined. Months later I heard from her again--it worked!

She'd not only had a fun, painless, blissful birth, but she actually experienced a truly orgasmic birth, like the ones I'd heard so much about but only seen one example of.

Yay! So it wasn't just a fluke. I now knew that I *could* pass on the information in a way that was successful in creating the change I wanted to create. At least one other woman had experienced the kind of birth I knew to be possible.

Even better, that mom was so excited about her birthing experience that she became a pregnancy coach and started spreading the word on her own.

The movement was officially born, and the secrets to blissful labor were on their way to reaching as many women as possible.

Chapter 16

Baby #3

Ben and Elizabeth had both heard the story of our trip to Santa Barbara, so from time to time they would ask if Baby Freedom were living in my belly yet. They both wanted another sibling to play with.

However, we were attempting "child-led weaning" with Elizabeth. My husband felt that I'd weaned Ben too early, at 2 years and 4 months.

At the time I was newly pregnant with Elizabeth and my breasts were extra tender. I *wanted* to wait for child-led weaning, but he showed no sign of ever slowing down. Fortunately, I had already night-weaned him, so that made it easier for him to adjust.

With Elizabeth, I'd agreed to let her nurse as long as she wanted... up to a point. I felt that her 4th birthday was plenty long enough, so I told her months in advance and she was mentally and emotionally prepared for the transition.

We night-weaned her right around 3½ years old, and I actually expected to get pregnant with baby #3 right away. After all, we'd gotten pregnant with

69

Elizabeth the very next month after night-weaning Ben.

Sure enough, the month after we transitioned to no night feedings for our little girl, we were pregnant again.

Pregnancy number three brought new experiences, and we went even more DIY than we had for Elizabeth's birth. We bought an inflatable kiddie pool on Amazon for $30 instead of renting an official water birth tub for over $300. Frugality really turns me on.

I found a blog post that listed out exactly what you need for a home water birth without any extra fluff. We ordered a water pump, faucet adapter, fish aquarium net to scoop out any debris that falls in the water, etc. Just the essentials.

On the Sunday morning two days before my official due date, I lost my "plug" while peeing. Hubby and I started to get excited.

The Braxton-Hicks contractions I'd been experiencing for weeks continued, but no other signs pointed to imminent labor. So we went through with our usual Sunday routine at the time.

We went to church, then dropped the kids off at Gramma & Grampa's so we could go on an afternoon date.

Since we knew the baby was coming soon, we decided to go for a walk at Descanso Gardens for our last just-the-two-of-us date. (You may remember that's where I was thinking about going right before I birthed Elizabeth.) We walked and talked and enjoyed the beauty of a mild February day in Southern California.

Then we picked up the kids and headed back home, where I made all the final preparations for birth. That evening, the Braxton-Hicks got closer and closer together.

I had a feeling the baby was coming, but since there were never any "intense" contractions, we weren't sure whether or not to fill up the kiddie pool. We didn't want the water to get cold if this was just the beginning of labor.

I just kept dancing and folding laundry and going about my evening, and the mini-contractions kept coming.

Finally I had my husband fill up the tub halfway just in case. And since it really could happen even faster, with the contractions so close together, I had him first fill up the giant Rubbermaid storage bin that the kids sometimes splash around in on a hot day.

The bin was pretty tiny for a pregnant woman, but there was just enough room for me to climb in and squat to have the baby if I needed to.

Having only ever experienced water births, I didn't want to try a "land birth," and the bin would only take a couple minutes to fill.

My body continued to tell me ever so gently that it was time for the baby to come. Hubby and I both had a hard time believing it, since I was so calm and the contractions were barely having any effect on me whatsoever. But I climbed into the tub anyway and started to really get into labor.

Chapter 17

Birthing Freedom

Since I'd learned even more about orgasmic birth since Elizabeth was born, I really wanted to see what that was like.

I thought it would be more likely to happen if I were feeling sexually aroused [*see the bonus chapter in the appendix for more on this*], but I just couldn't seem to flip that switch.

It didn't help that the inflatable kiddie pool was decorated with cartoon turtles and fish watching me with goofy bug-eyed grins. I tried closing my eyes and thinking erotic thoughts.

I even tried getting my husband in on the act [*for more detail on that part of the story, see my uncensored (and definitely "rated R for sexuality") video "**Stand Up Comedy Birthing Stories**" at **www.LoveBirthing.co**].*

However, once Freedom was ready to be born, he came so fast there wasn't even time for my body to interpret the sensations. The fetal ejection reflex kicked in quite suddenly, with no transition period or warning whatsoever.

Suddenly I was thrown back in the tub, and the baby's head crowned.

What I noticed right away was that there was a bunch of brown stuff floating in the water with me. In horror, I realized what it was.

"Grab the net!" I shrieked.

Ian had to find the net, scoop the "debris" out of the tub, and transfer it to the toilet.

Releasing all of the, um, debris in your body, in full view of everyone present at your birth (even if--or especially if--that's just your husband), is *not* one of my favorite parts of birthing.

Why during such a holy and beautiful moment?!

Anyway, one more FER rush and his little head was out. I could feel that the cord was wrapped around his neck, something I was prepared for after reading hundreds of birthing stories. I tried to gently unwrap it myself, but there wasn't enough slack for me to make it budge.

In my own memory of the moment, I panicked and freaked out about it and shouted frantically to my husband to help me. When I talked to him about it afterward, he assured me that I handled it like a pro.

I actually had to watch the birth video before I could believe him.

Sure enough, the video is almost completely silent. I whispered to hubby about the cord, he replied very calmly and quietly that I could handle it on my own, and I did.

The kids had been watching a Disney movie in the kitchen with Great Gramma and hadn't heard a thing. I sent Ian in to tell them their baby brother was here.

Freedom had come into the world so quietly that no one else in the house even knew I was in labor.

We let Elizabeth cut the cord this time, since Ben had gotten to cut hers. We harbored no fantasies of attempting a lotus birth, so we tied off the cord and cut it shortly after it stopped pulsing.

That made that first hour after birth so much easier. Ian and the kids were able to hold the baby a lot sooner, and I was able to get out of the tub on my own, clean up, and dry off.

When I sensed that the placenta was ready to come, I just squatted over a waterproof pad in the bathroom, and out it came. Simple enough.

But when I went to wrap the placenta in the pad, it sprang a leak. A pool of dark blood spread out from it and overflowed onto the bathroom floor faster than I could catch it.

Cleaning sticky blood off the bathroom linoleum isn't the kind of work I want to be doing right after giving birth. Next time maybe I'll deliver the placenta into a giant bowl.

So there it is, my birthing story so far (baby #4 is on the way as I type). All in all, Freedom's was another fantastic birth. Fun, fast, easy, and painless, leaving me even more convinced and eager to share the good news of blissful birthing with the world.

Appendix 1

What *IS* the Partner's Role Then?

While midwives and doulas can make great labor coaches, the birthing mother's partner is better suited to be her **advocate and guardian**.

You've most likely talked about how you'd prefer the birth to play out. You may not be in a place to communicate your wishes once you're deep in labor, so your partner can be your greatest ally.

Your partner can be the one fighting for you, staying firm for you, protecting you. That way you can relax and stay in the process of labor and delivery.

Staying relaxed and calm during labor is essential for achieving a truly natural birth.

Your partner can also help to keep the birthing environment calm and relaxing by paying attention to lighting, music, and the energy of those present.

Those are not details you want to be worrying about when you're in the midst of one of the most intense experiences of your life.

Let your partner be your protective guardian, kindly but firmly enforcing your choices, your wishes, and your boundaries, and being a loving supportive presence at your birth.

Appendix 2

Oversupply + What NOT to Do with Early Breastfeeding

Like many first-time mothers, I was concerned about my baby getting enough milk. I did everything I could to increase my supply, including drinking special herbal teas.

I also followed the recommendation that I feed my son for 15 minutes on each breast at each feeding. If he fell asleep while nursing, I even tickled his feet or chin to keep him awake enough to feed.

And it worked! My midwife was so impressed by his rapid growth and weight gain that she waived our 2-week postpartum checkup.

[*Note: We had also practiced a ton of skin-to-skin time, which is also known to support newborn weight gain and is often prescribed for preemies*].

Hooray! Full success! … Or was it?

Right at about the two-week mark, my precious little boy started to spit up after every feeding. And I don't just mean a little bit of milk, the amount that burp cloths were created to catch.

My tiny little guy would *projectile vomit* all over the place *after every feeding.*

I had to change his clothes, my clothes, the bedding, and anything else that had been hit. I started to keep a bucket next to me during feeding, which made cleanup way easier.

And I started to research like crazy. Was he allergic to something I was eating?

I went on a strict elimination diet to find out, reducing my menu options to plain potatoes, pears, plain turkey, and a few other very simple ingredients. I went *without chocolate* for two whole weeks!

The signs seemed to point to reflux, so we took all the steps we felt comfortable with (we're not quick to resort to pharmaceuticals).

We built him an incline ramp to sleep on. We massaged his tummy (not immediately after a feeding, of course). I drank lots of chamomile tea, hoping that would help his upset stomach.

But it wasn't until I was researching the next step of treatment that I stumbled upon the real root cause of our problem.

I'd heard that sucking on a pacifier could help create more saliva, which can calm a baby's tummy. But I'd also heard that offering a newborn a pacifier could cause nipple confusion and interfere with breastfeeding.

So I reached out to La Leche League International. They have a free online help form that allows you to ask any question and receive answers and support from a trained La Leche League leader.

I wanted to know which brand or type of pacifier they recommended for my situation--which one would cause the least amount of nipple confusion?

The reply really surprised me. The leader assigned to my question had seen too many cases of misdiagnosed infant reflux. She sent me a link to an article on La Leche League's website about "Oversupply," which I'd never even heard of.

It turned out Ben's "reflux" symptoms also matched those associated with oversupply of breastmilk. It wasn't that the milk was upsetting his tummy; he was just getting way too much of it!

The La Leche League leader then guided me to resources that helped me bump down my milk supply (feeding on only one breast for a certain number of hours, then switching to only the other breast, etc.) and we gradually got it all sorted out.

I've heard of reflux-diagnosed babies--*babies!*-- getting surgery to have their stomach flaps fixed, and their mothers having to wait helplessly as their little one undergoes this traumatic procedure.

If sharing my oversupply story helps just one family avoid that kind of unnecessary stress, I'll be happy.

Bonus Chapter

Orgasmic Birth/Get Yours Now (OB/GYN)

Most women I know wouldn't even want an orgasmic birth. The thought of it sounds distasteful or at least embarrassing.

They're planning on birthing with at least a midwife, if not their entire family and a team of doctors and nurses. So experiencing an orgasm in front of those people would be humiliating. I get that.

Or they believe that while of course it's normal, appropriate, and even preferable to orgasm while getting pregnant, it would be inappropriate to experience an orgasm at the moment of becoming a mother.

Got it. No problem with the logic in either case. Hey, I was raised in the church too. I know how absolutely taboo and fraught with deep emotions this whole conversation is.

However, I know there are at least a few women who actually *do* think that an orgasmic birth sounds like a beautiful experience, and who would love to know how they can increase their own chances of having one. It is for those women I've included this bonus chapter.

While some women purposely take their birth in an erotic direction in order to use pleasure as a tool for labor, that's certainly not a requirement for experiencing orgasm during delivery.

Many women have reported being completely surprised by the waves of pleasure that arrive out of nowhere and only later realize the only fitting label for them is "orgasmic." So orgasmic birthing does *not* necessarily mean sexually charged birthing.

The way I see it, there are **7 Key Steps to Having an Orgasmic Birth**.

1. *Want* an Orgasmic Birth.
2. Arrange for your labor to be as private as lovemaking.
3. Saturate your mind with pleasureful mantras and birthing stories.
4. Go completely *au natural* with your birth (drugs make it impossible).
5. Breathe and move like a vixen, moaning, panting, *feeling*....
6. Expecting pleasure, *slow... it... down.*
7. Enjoy whatever happens.

Of course, making orgasmic birth your *goal* could create unnecessary tension and actually reduce your chances of enjoying your birth experience fully.

It's no different than sex with orgasm as the goal-- never quite as good as just being there in the moment with the one you love.

No two births are exactly the same. So just enjoy the process, trust your body, and embrace the wild unpredictability of this once in a lifetime experience.

About the Author

AMANDA GRACE HARRISON is the creator of the **LoveBirthing Revolution**. After experiencing one traumatic "natural" birth and two blissfully painless unassisted home water births, she embarked on a mission to help make fun + easy labor the new normal for women around the globe.

A certified Laughter Yoga leader, Amanda loves dark chocolate, fresh flowers, bright colors, and great movies. She and her husband were married on a reality show (no, they didn't get matched up--it was the show *For Better or for Worse* on TLC, where a team of family and friends plan a surprise wedding for under $5k) and currently live in Los Angeles with their three (soon to be 4) kids.

What's next? Writing the *How to LOVE Birthing* handbook, giving birth to baby #4, making a documentary about *Blissful Birth*, co-writing a screenplay for *Sisterhood of the Traveling Birth Tub* (working title), taking a magical road trip adventure to share the books and films at screenings across the country…. Don't miss out on any of the exciting action!

Join the revolution and find out how YOU can be a part of the tribe changing the world together at **www.LoveBirthing.co**!

One Last Thing…

If you enjoyed this book or found it useful, I'd be soooooo grateful if you'd post a short review on Amazon. Your support really does make a difference. More positive reviews means more women will take a chance on reading the book. I also read each and every review personally so I can get your feedback and make this book even better.

Thanks so much for your support of the **LoveBirthing Revolution**.

Together, we're changing the world! :)

Made in the USA
Monee, IL
14 April 2022